A

MW01515603

Into the Night is Gary Barnes' thrilling story of facing death and disability and overcoming them both. Read it to ignite your courage, strengthen your resolve and show you the way to overcome your own tough times.

   – James Malinchak, Featured on
      ABC's hit TV show, "Secret Millionaire"
      Founder, www.BigMoneySpeaker.com

You have a story, a challenge...Gary's story will give yours perspective; make you laugh when you think you should be crying, cry when you're cheering him on and most importantly, make you realize that the only way to ever lose is to give up. What a powerful reminder to never, never, ever quit.

   Stunningly powerful, painfully personal, Gary shares his story of devastating challenge with a humor and levity that makes you love and respect him--displaying such grace and courage amidst the darkness that his remarkable rise back to Strength seems as much a given as it is against the odds. Gary's story of strength and courage, of love and compassion will help you see the strength in you to face whatever challenge you invite to your life and come through it freer, stronger and more alive.

   I am a better, more resourced man for having read Gary's story. Thank you for sharing your amazing strength with everyone.

   – Shawn Phillips - Founder at FULL Strength
      Nutrition, LLC, Fitness and nutrition veteran, for-
      merly of EAS fame, www.FullStrength.com

Into the Night captures one man's story of courage to defy death and disability. Captivating and thrilling, Gary's story is a must read that will inspire you to embrace destiny!'

– Avtar Nordine Zouareg - former Mr.Universe, Weight Loss and Wellness Guru, Best Selling Author, www.AvtarWellness.com

Thank you Gary for telling your story, as someone who also has been through similar adversities in my life your book is another great reminder of how powerful a positive attitude can be. Giving up is never an option, while finding the strength and courage to break through those limitations and face them head on is the best advice and a great reminder to us all.

– Brian Traichel - Director of Business Development at Brian Tracy International. FREE Brian Tracy Audio CD's http://budurl.com/BTFREE

Gary Barnes' new book *Into the Night* is a wonderful journey of perseverance and hope. Gary invites you to walk with him on his "adventure" into the world of MS. After every chapter you get action steps that you can apply to your journey that will help you move toward your goals. A truly inspirational book that you can't put down.

– Andrea Vahl (aka Grandma Mary) – Author, Speaker and Faccbook expert, www.AndreaVahl.com

Into the Night is not just a personal journey of a single man but a *human* journey—a guideline for all. It's an inspiration to follow your intuition, travel your own course and above all believe that nothing is impossible! How wonderful to see proof that the human experience can truly be limitless!

– Linda A. LeFebvre - Program Manager, Quality of Account Management

Knowing you personally, it was hard for me to hear in detail about the initial meetings with the doctors and the tests. I felt pain for you and what you were going through.

However, the raw courage you were able to muster to turn "like an eagle does" into the storm, engage the problem, own your results and ultimately take them in your hand to deliver your story for the benefit of others is exceptional.

I recommend this book to anyone who is thinking more about giving in than they are getting on. Gary's story is a vital reminder that we do have a powerful hand in our results despite very distressing circumstances, but we cannot count on things changing over night or wish our challenges away. However, we can count on the process of continuing to move forward with courage and a vision - a path that will lead to triumph.

– Marshall Foran - Author, Motivational Speaker,
  High Performance Coach,
  www.peakchievmentcoaching.com

TOTALLY engaging! I couldn't put it down! The Action Steps at the end of each chapter provide an immediate relationship to how Gary's stories pertain to OUR lives. His foundational blueprint shares how to remove the roadblocks in our lives, challenging us to see from a different perspective so that we may "triumph" and live the life of our dreams! I can instantaneously think of at least 5-10 people who need a copy of this "soul touching" chronicle. Thank you, Gary – so many of us needed this!

– Sallie Meshell - Author, Speaker, Trainer,
  www.DestinyByDesign.net

Gary Barnes' story is one of courage and determination. The focus and will he has developed through adversity is an example of how all of us can conquer any obstacle. As a coach, Gary has been invaluable to my business and my family. Words do not allow me to speak highly enough of him.

– Michael Arnold – Nationwide consultant to CPA firms, Palmetto Partners LLC, www.palmettopartners.net

Into the Night is an amazing life story about the challenges Gary faced when he was diagnosed with of two life threatening illnesses. Gary's intuitive wisdom, honesty and candor shows that life can and should be lived to the fullest, no matter what your circumstances. Gary's great humor makes it an easy and enjoyable read even though he is discussing very heavy topics. I highly recommend *Into the Night* for anyone facing adversity and searching for super ideas and techniques to move forward.

– Janie Smith – Author, Coach, www.hopebeyondtrauma.com

Gary's story inspires us at many levels. Not only is there hope in the midst of great adversity. Even more, there is a way for all of us to envision—and create—a great future. Thank you, Gary, for taking us on this journey with you.

– Steve Johnsen - The Website Income Strategist, Cumulus Consulting, www.cumulus-consulting.com

Wow! This book, *Into The Night*, was such an affirmation to me! It is such a quick read, yet so compelling and thought provoking.

When I came to the end of the first chapter and saw the first question that was poised to me, it was an eye opener!

Gary, carries you away with the story, yet brings you back to help you create your own story.

I am honored to have read this book. For me, right now, knowing where I am going, tomorrow I can just take a confident step forward to make my mark on history. Thank you Gary, for such insight and for telling your story.

Wherever you are in life is where you are suppose to be. Put a plan together, then add some goals and get this book to write your story.

– Suzi Nelsen – Group Travel Expert, Speaker,
www.CountriesandCrossroads.com

In his book, *Into the Night*, Gary Barnes shares a story that made me weep with tears and shout with joy as I praised God for his faithfulness, and for each of humanity's small yet steady triumphs over challenges that come in life. Gary's ability to connect people to his life journey filled with challenges, laughter, and praise moved me to reexamine life and the journeys taken along the way. A story of struggle and consistent power to overcome difficult situations, Gary finds a unique way of engaging the hearts of his readers to their internal source of power, designed to move them from victim to victorious. This is a book of HOPE, JOY, PRAISE, and POWER…all designed to break down the walls of healing and restrictions. It is a glorious and encouraging read! This book is filled with both humor and hope, two ingredients designed to overcome adversity! A must read for anyone in any situation who needs to be inspired with a powerful roadmap to moving beyond status quo.

– Dr. Virginia D. Moody - Author/Speaker/Life &
Career Coach, Moody & Associates
www.moody-associates.com

Gary Barnes is a masterful "traction" coach and a man with a big heart and deep wisdom. His newest book, *Into the Night*, is an inspiring tale for anyone who is ready to move beyond their perceived limitations and create an amazing life. If you are looking for motivation and guidance to overcome fear, obstacles and naysayers, you need to read this book.

> – Shannon Jackson Arnold - speaker and author of Flowering Wisdom: Inspiring Thoughts on Life, Love and Blooming Big,
> www.shannonjacksonarnold.com

Gary truly takes the reader *Into the Night* as his companion on a long walk from a snowy day 22 years ago and a life-changing diagnosis to a future no less uncertain than that of anyone else. And what an amazing journey it is. Told in his own words (truly!), Gary shares the reality, the emotion, the resolution, and the process by which he faced down a medical death sentence and chose to turn it into a life sentence. *Into the Night* is much more than a personal memoir—Gary's story is an inspirational gift that holds lessons for each of us to find and embrace.

> – CaZ...Candy Zulkosky, www.myTechDiva.com

So heartfelt and moving. Love your sense of humor and how you share your experience, thoughts and feelings, then let us, the readers, know what you decided to do and the action steps you took to over come the obstacles and challenges you faced. Then after all that, you give us questions to help us think and work through our own obstacles and challenges!

> – Tori Underwood – Business Development Consultant, www.torilynnconsulting.com

To Live is exactly what Gary does every day, this means that the laughter, joy and of course a few obstacles never ends. Challenges are just opportunities to grow and learn, either you can or you cannot, will or you will not, there is no try! Gary proves that he controls his mind—his mind does not control him. This book shares a journey that will ask you what you are doing with your 24-hour deposit. Will you be a participant or spectator? *Into the Night* will provide you with a wealth of information to embrace your journey.

– Gale Neiderworder - Kairos Center for Healing
www.denverhealing.com

Gary shares a poignant journey of the strength and perseverance it takes to overcome adversity. His detailed recount of the events brings us along on his painful, scary and bewildered path but he doesn't just leave us there. He also brings us along with his wonderfully-gifted sense of humor. This humor somehow lessens the pain and helps to put the whole picture into a better perspective. I love how he refuses to accept the destiny that others defined for him and that he chooses to live life fully in spite of the challenges. His creative visualization technique is inspiring (and better yet, defied the odds for improving his health)! You must read this story and let Gary inspire you to face your challenges head on while living life with a zest and zeal that is so 'Gary'. He inspires me and he is sure to inspire you too.

– Karen Schatz, Virtually With You Virtual Assistance,
www.VirtuallyWithYou.com

By sharing *Into the Night*, Gary gives us the gift of belief, hope, and positivity, so that we are clear that we have the right to determine the course of our lives in order to pursue the happiness that we dream, desire, and deserve. Gary has taught me: a diagnosis is just someone else's opinion, and that your life purpose need be your only truth.

– Andrea Adams-Miller - Leading Authority in
  Healthy Relationships & Healthy Sexuality,
  www.SexualityTutor.com &
  www.AndreaAdams-Miller.com

Don't read this book if you like feeling sorry for yourself and want others to join you in this small game. Gary Barnes says there is another way to play the game of life, one that enlarges the playing field, even when life deals unpleasant surprises. How can you make that shift? Gary tells his own compelling story of adversity overcome; even better, he tells us what questions to ask in our own stories to find a bigger game. I have found them useful as I travel life's road with a cancer diagnosis. I'm not giving in to a small world experience.

– Glenn Sackett - Glenn Sackett Photography,
  www.GlennSackett.com

Into the Night is one of those inspirational books that's filled with messages that stick with you long after you've finished reading. By sharing his story, Gary demonstrates that we all make choices in our lives every day. As he points out, everyone deals with adversity; it's how you react to the adversity that can change the "adventure" that is your life. In this moving book, Gary explains how he created his own "road to success" and offers insights into how you can realize the vision you have for your life too.

– Susan Daffron (aka The Book Consultant)
  President. Logical Expressions, Inc.
  www.LogicalExpressions.com

Into the Night

The Road from Adversity to Triumph

Gary Barnes

Dedication

It has been said that no man is an island and that is very true for my life. First and foremost I want to dedicate this book to my wife Sharon, who has chosen to walk my story with me for the last 37 years. To my children Matt and Kelly, Chris and Abby, and Jason and Desiree Sornsuwan. You all have supported me in a way that has been and still is extraordinary.

Thank you Matt and Kelly Barnes and Sharon for all of your work in the editing of this book. Thank you also Jason for the phenomenal book cover design! (www.sornsuwanphotography.com)

Thank you Susan Daffron (www.logicalexpressions.com) for all of the handholding in getting this first physical book out. Even though I am self-publishing, I feel like you are truly my publisher and mentor.

There are also many who have encouraged me to capture my story in a book form, and I thank you all.

Contents

Introduction

Why did I write this book? Because I never actually intended to. I know we all have adversity that comes into our lives, and I didn't think my story was all that special. However, because of those who have heard my story and urged me to share it in a book, I have finally relented.

I believe everyone that has overcome adversity is special and every person, at sometime in their life, will be faced with adversity. It is our response to adversity that will determine our ultimate results, not the adversity itself. The adversity is only the trigger and stimulus. I am not promising any special formula or a magic bean to plant that will make all of your challenges disappear. What I will do is share my experiences as they happened. I will also share the process, tools, and techniques that I used to create an unusual outcome according to the professionals that dealt with me.

As you read this book, my hope is that you don't read it as a spectator but rather as someone who is walking beside me in my journey. You will have opportunities at the end of each chapter to reflect and respond to questions I have asked you to look at, as they might apply to your life.

Over the years I have come to embrace the idea that I'm not looking for better answers. I am looking for better questions that lead me to an answer, which will lead me to another better question. As I receive answers to a question it only becomes my reality if I accept the answer as fact. That's why one of my Gary-isms is to "question reality." You will have a better understanding of this concept as you read my story, for if I had accepted the doctor's answers as facts regarding the condition I faced, I would not be here to write this book. I would simply have been another statistic and memory in the lives of my family, friends, and clients.

I would also like to invite and encourage anyone who would like to reach out to me with a question, or if you would just like to share your story with me, to do so. You will find my contact information at the back of this book.

I see this as an adventure. The final chapter has yet to be written, but I will share with you the events on the road I have lived for the last 22 years.

1

A Twist in the Road

As we approached the Thanksgiving weekend of 1988 we experienced a late fall snowstorm that was heavy with water content. For anyone that does not live in snow country, what this means is the snow is very heavy to shovel. My wife, Sharon, and I had moved our sons, Matt and Chris, in 1984 from Southern California to Denver, Colorado. I was still getting used to the changing of the seasons and, while it was enjoyable, shoveling snow was not one of my most enjoyable activities.

I decided to get a head start on clearing the driveway before the boys got home from school. About halfway through the job I picked up a particularly heavy shovelful of snow. I immediately felt a sharp jabbing pain in the palm of my right hand. I rubbed the spot and the pain subsided, so I continued to shovel the snow. By the time I finished clearing the driveway, I noticed a numbness crawling up my right arm. I remember thinking to myself this was not normal, but I figured it would get better all by itself.

> *I remember thinking to myself this was not normal, but I figured it would get better all by itself.*

Within the next hour and a half the numbness radiated up my arm, across my chest, and down my left side.

Having never experienced something like this before, I wondered if I had pinched a nerve in my neck or back when I was shoveling the very heavy wet snow. Because of the numbness from the neck down, I also noticed that I was losing a little bit of my coordination. I didn't want to alarm my wife and family, so I decided to keep it to myself and see how I felt in the morning. I know it can be somewhat of a guy thing, but somehow I thought if I would just ignore the symptoms it would all get better.

When I woke up the next morning I felt fine. I started to do an inventory of all my body parts and they all seemed to be working. Encouraged by my insightfulness and not sharing the previous day's events with the family I jumped out of bed, and that's when the real adventure began. As soon as my feet hit the floor I fell flat on my nose (I remember thinking to myself this was not a good situation). It happened so quickly that it caught me completely by surprise. It also startled my wife, but by this time in our marriage she knew that I was always clowning around. She asked me what I was doing down there and I had to come clean about what happened the day before.

One of the reasons that we moved to Colorado was that Sharon had a job opportunity at one of the major hospitals in the area. I feel fortunate because she had access to the medical community in a quick way. I'm the typical type of person that only goes to a doctor when they think they are dying. My experience with doctors is that they rarely give you good news. Sharon wanted me to see a doctor right away, and although I didn't want to admit it I was a little scared. We called our primary care doctor and were able to get an appointment immediately.

When I arrived for my appointment I was still fully confident that I had just pinched a nerve in my neck, and that he would tell me to take it easy and maybe give me a muscle relaxer and send me on my way. I was way too busy to take time out of my calendar and wanted a quick fix.

My initial exam was quick, but instead of sending me home with a prescription, he sent me directly to a neurologist whose office was in the same medical building. This increased my level of concern, because when you go see a specialist it doesn't mean that you are special; it means that you may become a reference in a medical journal at some point. I knew, though, that it was important for me to find out what was happening to my body, so upstairs I went.

Now I hope I don't offend any neurologists that may read my story, but anyone that has seen a neurologist knows they like to pinch and poke. Even though by this time I had lost all of the feeling from my neck down, fell on my nose, and saw the concerned look on my primary care doctor's face, I still believed what was happening to me was nothing serious. The neurologist conducted what I considered very low-tech medical techniques. He asked me to close my eyes and then to put my forefinger on my nose. I never really excelled at taking tests, but this one was a no-brainer—I could do this! I wanted to show this doctor that I was in complete control of my body and promptly put my finger in my ear. Now knowing this was not the desired outcome I slowly moved my finger across my cheek and up on my nose. Maybe the doctor hadn't noticed. As I looked up, I saw the stern look of the doctor that said that I had cheated and he had caught me.

Strike one!

He then wanted me to walk in a straight line, just like you would if you were taking a sobriety test. Again I thought to myself, fantastic, I can redeem myself. I have been walking a straight line since I was about 12 months old. He laid out my path and told me to start. The moment I took my first step I could've sworn we were experiencing an earthquake, because the floors seemed to move in a different direction every time I took a step. The harder I focused on directing my body to go a certain way, the more it rebelled and went another.

Rats--strike two!!

He then took out a medical instrument that resembled an old-fashioned pinwheel. It had sharp points and was round (why do medical instruments look like something you would find in a medieval castle torture chamber?). Then he said he was going to roll it up my arms, legs, and feet. Okay, here's a test that I couldn't fail because I didn't even have to move. Then he put in another twist to the test—I had to close my eyes and tell him where he was rolling the pointy little instrument. I think I even saw him smile a little as he said it.

As he began asking where he was poking me, the macho side of me showed up. I knew that I had failed the first two tests and didn't want to strike out, so I did what any red blooded male would—I guessed. It didn't take long for him to figure out what I was doing, because he would poke my leg and I would say he poked my foot. I think by this time I figured out my self-diagnosis of a pinched nerve was not going to be his diagnosis.

Strike three!!! OK Coach, where is the dugout?

He said that even though it was a holiday week he wanted me to take a fairly new test called an MRI. There was only one location in the state of Colorado, but he would see what availability he could get for me to take the test as soon as possible. He then left me in the exam room for me to think about my predicament. My immediate thought was if only I had not gone out to shovel the snow I would not be wasting my time now in a doctor's office. I had always been active playing sports and had received some injuries, but I could always see the direct cause. This was something different.

My personality is if I'm facing a challenge; just tell me what to do. I felt like I was fighting an invisible enemy, but I still believed that I wasn't dealing with anything all that serious.

> *I felt like I was fighting an invisible enemy*

When the doctor returned, he had an appointment in hand. He had pulled some strings and made the appointment for me to have an MRI completed at 11 PM on the Saturday night of Thanksgiving weekend. I told him that I appreciated all of his hard work, but can we do this after the holidays? It was then that I had my first real look at the seriousness of my situation. He sat quietly for what seemed like an eternity, but finally looked up at me and he said, "Gary, there are three choices in what you're dealing with. You may have cancer, a brain tumor, or Multiple Sclerosis."

> *You may have cancer, a brain tumor, or Multiple Sclerosis. I didn't like those three choices*

I didn't like those three choices and being sort of a wise butt at times, I looked straight back at him and said, "No thanks, I would like what's behind door number four." He looked at me like I was a little crazy and said, "Let's just see what the test results say."

So with that encouraging start to my new adventure I went home to "enjoy" the Thanksgiving Holiday with my family.

Action Steps Chapter 1

At the end of each chapter, as we take this journey together, I thought it would be beneficial to you, the reader, if I would ask a question that you can apply to your own life situation. So here's your first one.

We each have our own personal story. The question that I would like to ask you to ponder first is, what is your story? At this time you don't have to capture all of the details; just do a quick outline. Second, what adversity have you experienced in your life or are currently experiencing? Identify specifically what the challenges are, although it is not necessary right now to look for a solution.

Thanks for playing!

2

The Machine

To say the least, Thanksgiving was a little different that year. We didn't talk much about what
I was going through, except for the fact that I was
having difficulty walking. I believe this was because
we didn't know what I was facing, and I was still
looking for that door number four option.

By the time Saturday came I knew it would not
be wise for me to drive myself to the MRI exam. I
didn't have any feelings in any of my extremities from
the neck down and driving at night, in that condition, would be dangerous. I knew Sharon wanted
to go, but I didn't want to be dependent on anyone

for my mobility. It has been my custom when we go somewhere together that I always drive. The thought of losing that independence was disturbing. I was also concerned about taking the MRI exam. What was it going to show? According to the professionals, the MRI was going to indicate whether it was cancer, a brain tumor, or Multiple Sclerosis, so there was no positive outcome.

MRIs in 1988 were totally brand-new, so I didn't know what to expect. The neurologist had said it was no big deal, and all I had to do was lay still and let the machine do all the work. So here I am again, another test. I had struck out with the three tests the doctor had already given me in his office. Now I had an opportunity to redeem myself.

I remember it being very cold that evening as we drove south of Denver to where the MRI testing site was located. As we drove up to the facility I was expecting to enter a medical building full of well-meaning people. What we found instead was an 18 wheeler tractor trailer that had been converted into an MRI exam room. WOW, I thought to myself this really **is** new.

When we entered the trailer we were greeted by a technician. A young woman who seemed very pleasant was reassuring. I was advised to make absolutely sure that I had nothing metallic in my pockets because the MRI basically is a huge magnet. If I inadvertently left anything metallic on my clothing, it would be ripped through my clothing and would stick to the side of the MRI machine. She then had me take off my shirt and gave me a hospital gown to put on (if there are any clothing designers reading this, would it be too much to ask to have you design a hospital gown that was flattering?).

When I was duly prepared, the technician escorted me into the exam room to meet "the machine." When I first looked at it, it had the appearance

> *When I was duly prepared, the technician escorted me into the exam room to meet "the machine."*

of a science-fiction Time Machine. It had a stainless steel table that was on rollers. It resembled one of the cadaver tables I had seen in my college biology lab. A pleasant thought! She asked me to lie down on the table face up. Then she positioned my head on a formed pillow type of object and told me that I could not move my head during the test. If I did move the pictures would be blurry, and I would have to do it all over again. She also explained that during the exam the MRI would be extremely loud. She said it was a sound that was a cross between machine-gun fire and someone hammering rapidly on a piece of metal.

She asked if I was ready to start the exam, without really knowing what I was saying yes to, I said, "Sure, let the fun begin." She again reassured me that taking the test was nothing to be afraid of. If I needed anything during the exam, all I had to do was to call out to her and she would hear me.

Now taking an MRI exam is a unique experience. If you have had the pleasure of taking an MRI you know what I mean. I was lying on the table and she proceeded to push me literally head first into the machine. As I looked up, the enclosure where my head was started to get smaller and smaller. I had never felt claustrophobic before, but as I went further and further into the machine, and as the space between my nose and the top of the cylinder got closer, I started to sweat a little. At last she had me positioned correctly and, as I looked up, it seemed that there was only about an inch from the tip of my nose to the bottom of the machine. It was then I knew for sure that this was going to be an interesting experience.

The technician spoke to me through a speaker and said we were ready to start and again encouraged me to lie perfectly still. Most of the time I would have come back with a smart aleck retort, but this time I knew I wanted to be good, so I wouldn't have to retake this crazy test.

Wow, when she said that the noise of the MRI was loud she wasn't kidding. It was like they were testing my ability not to jump out of my skin when the test started. There were four sections to the exam, and I knew right away that I had to create some sort of diversion for me to take my mind off the noise and the extremely small space I found myself in. I decided to take a little trip. I love the ocean, and Sharon and I had taken a vacation to Hawaii a few years before, so I decided to relive that trip. I visualized walking along the beach, feeling the ocean breeze and enjoying paradise. To my relief it worked, and I relaxed as much as I think anyone could in that situation.

After the first two tests, I thought I would check and see if the technician had told me the truth about her availability if I needed her. So I called out her name. No response. A bead of sweat started to form on my forehead. I called again. Still no response! Now what? A little feeling of panic started to creep into my consciousness. Was the speaker just not working? Had she taken a break, or was she just playing a practical joke on me? I have a pretty good imagination, and now it started to work overtime. I was alone, in the middle of the night, and in a machine that I was growing to dislike with every passing minute.

I had to fight the feeling that I had to escape from the bowels of this machine before it was too late.

I had to fight the feeling that I had to escape from the bowels of this machine before it was too late. But, too late for what? I decided to give it another go and called out her name again. To my relief she said,

"Hi, Gary. What can I do for you?" I told her that I had been calling her name to test and see if she was really there. She said that she had stepped out for just a moment and was so sorry to cause any concern on my part. In all of the macho vibrato that I could muster I said, "No worries, I was just seeing if everything was working." I wonder if she knew?

As the technician completed the last two sections of the MRI, I again went back to my visualization of our trip to Hawaii. It really is amazing how vivid our imaginations can be. Here I was in a stressful situation, but my visualization was so real to me that it seemed I could hear the ocean and feel the warmth of the tropical breeze. Up to this point I had been focusing on taking the test itself and not on the results. Towards the end of this process the question of what the test results would reveal started to creep in. What was it going to show? Was it going to reveal that I had a terminal illness or some other form of disease that had catastrophic consequences? Somehow I knew I needed to stop the negative story making of my future. So, I figured I would look only at what my next step could be.

When I was finished with the exam the technician pulled me out of the machine. What a relief! I was free! I thought to myself "that wasn't so bad." Yeah right. So now what? When my technician (notice that she had become *my* technician not *the* technician. For the last hour and a half she had been my lifeline to the outside world) came in to sign me out I asked her, "What did the results look like?" She told me not to worry about that and my doctor would be in touch with me sometime next week after he had a good opportunity to review the test results. I started seeing a pattern in people telling me not to worry, and the more they told me not to worry the more concerned I got.

So off into the night Sharon and I went. Did I pass the test? We didn't talk much about the future on the way home. I was too busy sharing all of details of the adventure of the MRI itself. We both knew that this was the start of a major change in our lives.

Action Steps - Chapter 2

What tests are you facing right now or did you face in the past in your relationships, in business, or any other area of your life? Especially look at any situation where the test results are totally unknown and out of your control.

There are no right or wrong answers. Please don't feel like you have to come up with a major test in order to get maximum benefit out of these action steps. If you're not able to connect with a personal test you can always come back at a later time when one shows up.

3

The Longest Night

It had been a very short night but with two young sons, sleeping in was not an option. It was quickly becoming my habit that when I woke up in the morning I would do an inventory of my body to see if it was just a really weird dream, and if I was back to normal. As I went through this exercise on that Sunday morning I knew that I had not gotten any better but, likewise, I was not any worse. A small victory.

The day was uneventful until that evening. Around eight o'clock the telephone rang, and when

I answered it I was very surprised to be greeted by the voice of my neurologist.

He told me in a very matter-of-fact way that he had reviewed the MRI results, and that he wanted to see my wife and me in his office at eight o'clock the next morning. Now I don't know about you, but if you receive a phone call from your doctor on a weekend, at 8 o'clock in the evening, and he wants you to be in his office and to bring your wife, basically in a few hours this can heighten your level of concern. On top of that I knew that Mondays were his days off. Not a good sign. I asked him what the test results showed, and he said he would cover all of that the next morning with my wife and me and "not to worry."

Again the "not to worry" statement. No problem, I just wanted to know what not to worry about!

> *No problem, I just wanted to know what not to worry about!*

As we finished up the day's chores and got the boys off to bed my mind again started to create a story of doom. We decided to go to bed early, since the previous night had been a short night, and we knew that Monday morning would more than likely be very stressful. As I settled in to go to sleep my mind just wouldn't shut off. I had gone through adversity before in my life but somehow this was different.

I started to think about all of the things I wanted to do. My sons were seven and nine years old. I wanted to see them graduate from high school and then college. I wanted to see them fall in love and get married, and I wanted to be a part of my grandchildren's lives—not just be a memory or someone that sat in a corner that they referred to as Grandpa. I wanted to be active and participate in everyone's lives.

And what about Sharon? We had been married 13 years by this time, but nothing had prepared us to handle a situation like this. This event had not been part of our plan. I knew I didn't want to be a burden on Sharon or the rest

> *Part of my mission statement is "to live life, not merely exist".*

of my family. Part of my mission statement is "to live life, not merely exist."

I kept going over all of what I thought would be the possibilities from the doctor's verdict tomorrow. Every time I would run down a scenario, the ending to the story was not very comforting. I finally drifted off into a very non-restful sleep.

Eight o'clock the next morning found us in the neurologist's office. His nurse came out to greet us and brought us into an exam room. Sharon and I were not talking a lot, as I think we were both lost in our own wonderings. I soon became bored, however, and started looking around the room for something to play with that would occupy my time. I found one of those instruments that doctors use to hit your knee to see how well your reflexes are working and started do a test on myself. Before Sharon could say something about acting my age, the doctor came in with what looked like x-ray film. He started out by thanking us for coming in on such short notice, but he wanted us to have the results of my MRI as quickly as possible.

Remember at the end of my first appointment with the neurologist, he had given me three choices of what the situation was. The possibilities were a brain tumor, cancer, or Multiple Sclerosis. Over the years I have found that doctors really dislike giving bad news to their patients, and he was no different, so for the next hour he explained in detail everything that wasn't wrong with me. My wife, also being a medical professional, wanted all of the specifics. I, being an expressive driver personality, wanted the bottom line and to determine what our course of action was going to be. (When I went on road trips as a kid, my favorite question was "are we there yet?")

Finally, I couldn't wait any longer. I said, "Doc, you've told us everything that it isn't; I need to know what the final results of the MRI are. What are we dealing with?" He looked down at his chart again, seemingly hesitant to share that knowledge. He finally looked up at me and said, "You still have three choices, but they're all the same. You have MS, MS, or MS." The room went silent as we took in this bit of news.

I quickly went back to the original three options, and it occurred to me that the doctor's diagnosis was actually a life sentence, not a death sentence. I had heard of Multiple Sclerosis before but didn't really know anything specific about the condition. My wife, however, in her first position out of graduate school, dealt with MS patients. She saw the outcomes and the processes for these people and knew that the future for us would have many challenges.

> *The doctor's diagnosis was actually a life sentence, not a death sentence*

Not knowing this information (which, by the way, I think helped me) I asked the doctor, "What do we do now?" He looked at me a little bewildered because I think he fully expected me to fall apart with the news. I told the doctor that I thought this was great because he had really given me a life sentence, and I wanted to know what our process was in order to meet this challenge head-on.

He told me that I wasn't really grasping the situation, that my options were limited. Maybe I could use steroids but the after-effects could be as debilitating as the illness itself. OK, then what was my second choice? I could tell by his expression that he thought I just wasn't getting it, that my option was that there was no option. I had to come to grips with the fact that my life had taken an unfortunate turn for the worst. It was his opinion that I would be in a wheelchair or dead within 10 years. I had to be realistic about what my future held.

At that moment something I can only refer to as my intuition kicked in. I knew instantly that if I ever said that I *had* something (MS) and *owned* the diagnosis the doctor had just given me, the prediction the doctor had just detailed would come true. Because of that intuitive moment, I have always said I was *diagnosed with* Multiple Sclerosis in 1988.

I still had all of the symptoms. At that time I could not write my name, feel anything from the neck down, walk a straight line or even walk without tripping, or accurately feed myself, but I knew if I ever accepted the diagnosis as fact that I would seal my doom.

I knew if I ever accepted the diagnosis as fact that I would seal my doom.

As a side note I believe that our intuition is that whisper or still small voice that we refer to as God, the infinite intelligence, source, or any other name that we attach to the higher power that's in control of this universe. Please do not mistake this explanation as an opportunity for me to share my spiritual beliefs. I only offer it as a possible insight to be used by anyone in a stressful situation. I believe that the only reason I'm here sharing my story with you is that I paid attention to my intuition that day.

I know the doctor was being very honest, and he was concerned about my seeming lack of acceptance of the severity of the situation. He was concerned that I didn't get my hopes up unrealistically. As we were wrapping up the appointment and got up to leave I wanted to give him a clear perspective of what my intentions were. I told him, "Doc, I truly don't know what the future holds, but I do know that I'm not waiting around for this illness. It's got to catch me!"

As we walked out of the medical building into the cool air of that November morning, what we just experienced still didn't seem real. It was a beautiful day with a brilliant blue sky that we often have here in Colorado. Could it be that it was only a week ago that my life seemed normal? What was our future going to be? My intuition was still telling me that it was going to be all right, but the fear was still there. I knew the fear came from the uncertainty of not knowing what the future held (as if we ever do) and not having a definitive plan to work from to receive an outcome that was acceptable to me.

I wanted a roadmap, a plan of action that would give me a fighting chance to beat the odds. Since the doctor had nothing to offer I was determined to create my own road to success.

I stumbled a little as I reached the car, which reminded me that the road ahead would, at times, be difficult. I also knew that the adventure of my life had just begun.

Action Steps - Chapter 3

I would like you to think about whatever particular situation you find yourself in. What is your plan of action? Again, this does not have to be extremely detailed. Using bullet points is totally fine. We're only looking for what your next one or two steps are going to be.

4

What Now? The Decision to Live!

So now what? Being reminded every moment that my body was not responding to my mind was extremely challenging. I knew the decisions I would be making in the next few weeks would have lifelong effects. I don't remember ever feeling sorry for myself or asking the proverbial "why me" question, but I do remember being angry. Angry at my body for betraying me. Angry at God for seemingly not caring about me. Angry at myself for somehow allowing this event to happen in my life. All very rational thoughts, I know.

As I was grasping to put the events of the last week or so into perspective the question occurred to me: Was this an adversity or a blessing? When I was at the doctor's office, and he told me of his diagnosis I was actually happy that he had given me—in my mind—a life sentence. Was that really true? Yes, he had given me a life sentence, but how could I see a blessing in all of the changes that were happening to me? Changes? Yes, they were changes, but they were losses as well.

> *Was this an adversity or a blessing?*

One of the feelings that developed early in this experience was that I was trapped in my body. The thought was that if somehow I could just break through this invisible barrier all of my feeling would come back. It was like I was falling into a deep hole without having anything to grab onto to stop my fall. Again I knew I had to stop focusing on my present condition.

Then a twist in my story happened. In my oldest son Matt's class there were three parents going through life-threatening situations. There were two mothers and myself. One of the mothers was dealing with a brain tumor, the other cancer. It seemed ironic to me that the three choices the neurologist had given me were the same three conditions we parents were dealing with. Matt's class took us all on as sort of a project. They wrote get well cards to all of us (and I still have them), giving us encouragement and hope for the future. As I read those cards and heard the stories of the two mothers, I realized I could embrace my situation as either an adversity or a blessing—it was truly my choice. I knew the choices were quantity of life and quality of life. I wanted both, but if I had to choose, I would choose quality of life. I made the conscious choice to focus on what I wanted my future to be and not on the fear of what it might be.

I have also always been the person who looks at any situation a little differently. I'll clown around, make jokes, and get away with it at times when others would get in trouble for doing the same thing. I noticed that when I went out in public people saw my unbalanced walk. Little children would sometimes point and say something to their parents, and they would look at me to see if I might be either drunk or crazy. I would see the parents shield their children as if I might somehow be a danger to their child.

This hurt, but I knew that being unusual or different in our society can be threatening. So I wanted to come up with something that I could say to bridge the gap. What I came up with was, "Hire the handicapped, we're fun to watch!" If you took a little gasp as you read my little saying you're not alone. This is not a self-deprecating statement but one, rather, to shine a bright light on the elephant in the room. At that time there was little I could do about the symptoms I was experiencing, but I could share with those around me and make a connection with humor.

> *"Hire the handicapped, we're fun to watch!"*

My boys also helped with this process of being "normal", while also being "different" than other people. As I mentioned, when I would feed myself many times my food would end up in a place other than in my mouth. As a routine I would also test myself with the finger to the nose trick to see if I was gaining my coordination back. As the boys watched, it soon became a game. We would be at the dinner table or in the car or just sitting around the house, and they would ask me to do the finger trick. They would even ask me to perform this feat for anyone they came in contact with. At the mall, in restaurants, it didn't really matter to them. Even though it was a simple little process, it really helped.

I knew I needed a concrete process and vision to be able to create all of the benefits this new life had to offer. I started to think about how long I was planning to live. I remembered reading a story about George Burns, the comedian. He was planning a very long and energetic life and believed in it so much that he booked himself to do a comedy show in Las Vegas on his 100th birthday. I thought this was very cool, and so I embraced the concept of living to 100. I also didn't want to just be alive until I was 100, I wanted to be active and vibrant, participating in life. What could I do to celebrate my 100th birthday? The answer was obvious, I would go skydiving! I got really excited about this thought of being 100 and jumping out of an airplane. I have always loved flying. It has been said that you have to ask yourself two questions before leaving a perfectly good aircraft. First, is the airplane broken? Second, can it be fixed? It is only with a "yes" and then a "no" answer do you ever consider jumping out of a perfectly good airplane. Notwithstanding this sage advice, I knew this would be my great adventure on my 100th birthday.

But what could I focus on now that would make a difference to me tomorrow, next week, or next month? In 1988 the concept of visualization was somewhat new. I had read the story of Norman Cousins ("Anatomy of an Illness") who had been diagnosed with Ankylosing Spondylitis, which is a condition in which the connective tissue in the spine deteriorates. He used what is now known as laugh therapy to put this very painful and debilitating illness into remission. He thought the Marx Brothers and Candid Camera were the funniest comics and real-life situations around and would spend hours and hours watching their movies. There were also stories of other people with the diagnosis of cancer that used the imagery of the little Pac-Man icons moving throughout their bloodstream gobbling up the bad cancer cells. To many this may seem silly and very nonscientific, but it worked for them.

Please don't misunderstand that I'm telling you not to use all of what the medical community has to offer. There are many medical professionals that are dedicated to those that are afflicted with an illness. As you will see in the next chapter I did not ignore the medical community, but the medical community did not have much to offer me in the way of process to change my outcome. I just wasn't ready to lay down and die, so I came up with an alternative.

In reading these stories, while they were inspiring, they did not really relate to my specific situation. I needed to come up with something that would directly give me a picture of my progress. Something that my expressive/driver personality could get excited about. I laid in bed thinking about what story I could create that would give me inspiration and hope. I thought about somehow using eagles as part of my visualization. Eagles have always been my favorite animal. They are one of the few animals that, when a storm approaches, turn into it, and face it head-on. I knew that was my attitude, but how could I directly connect what an eagle does and what I needed fixed in my body? Well, that didn't work, so what would be Plan B? That question would change my life forever. Almost immediately a picture of a beaver came into my mind. Of course a beaver, that was the answer! At this point you may think for sure I'm a little nuts and I may be, but this concept of a beaver working in my brain would have a result that has astounded every neurologist I have seen. The party begins!

Action Steps - Chapter 4

Make a list of all the things that make you normal and then make a list of all the things that make you different. Then look at the two lists to see where they connect. It's been my experience that where the two lists connect is how the outside world sees us. This can be very useful information in any situation.

5

My New "Best Friends"

When the news of my diagnosis reached our family and friends, I was inundated with their good intentions. It's only natural and normal for people to want to help out in any life changing situation. The challenge can be that their good intentions can be overwhelming. I think I received every article, book, diet plan, and new medical and alternative technique on how to deal with the diagnosis of MS. I am more doer than researcher, which also has its drawbacks, but I remembered reading stories of medical students manifesting the symptoms of whatever illness they happened to be studying at the time. That's not what I wanted to do. I just wanted to understand what happened in the brain to cause the effects of my experience.

So here is my elementary explanation of what happened in my brain that created the symptoms I experienced. I look at the brain as being a big battery. The nerves in the brain, then, are like electric wires. There is a coating around the nerves in our brains that keeps the raw nerves from touching each other. It's very much like the coating around an electric wire. For some reason this coating, called the myelin sheath, dissolves.

When the exposed nerves touch each other they short out the electrical signal that the nerve is carrying and cause a lesion. As the lesion heals it forms a scab over the site, effectively blocking any electrical signal that the nerve had been transmitting. Depending on where that nerve was connected, it virtually disrupts that bodily function. It is also believed that once a

> *So this was my problem, how could I rewire my brain?*

lesion has formed, and a scab has formed, it will never go away. So this was my problem, how could I rewire my brain? That's where my beaver friend came into play.

The connection to the beaver and a relevant visualization for me was the beaver's tail. I thought if the myelin sheath dissolved then it could be repaired. If it couldn't be repaired, I wanted it to be rewired. I figured that if any section of the nerve could not be repaired, I simply would have the beavers splice in wire going around the damaged area. I decided to visualize my new beaver friend in my brain as I was going to sleep each night. I lay in bed, and the beaver showed up for work. I specifically challenged him to start anywhere in my brain and when he found a break in the myelin sheath he was to repair it. I saw this beaver as being very energetic and confident, totally dedicated to one thing, redirecting those electrical impulses, so that I could regain my mobility and feeling.

I saw this beaver in my brain every single night, but I soon realized what an enormous job this would be for a single beaver. My expressive self had the answer, if one beaver is good two or more beavers are great. Over the next month or so I created a complete community of beavers in my brain. I had three full shifts of beavers working around the clock. There was a school, community center, stores, and housing developments (I wanted to take good care of my beavers and their families). We even had a recreation center.

With this new army of beavers solely focused on repairing my brain, I did not see any way that I would not experience improvement in my motor functions. I still could not write, walk a straight line, or do many of the seemingly menial tasks that even a young child could do, including buttoning my shirt or tying my shoes.

> *I knew instinctively that I needed to focus on where I wanted to go and not on my current experience.*

Again I knew instinctively that I needed to focus on where I wanted to go and not on my current experience. I would spend over two hours per night lying in bed, directing my beavers on what to do. In a very real sense they became my friends.

On one of my visits to the original neurologist I shared my visualization with him. He again advised me not to get my hopes up, and that while he didn't think that it would do me any harm, it probably would not give me any significant benefit either. There were times that I wanted to give up on my visualization, because I didn't see the immediate results I wanted.

I was experiencing pain and discomfort, sometimes feeling like my hands and feet were going to explode. I would get itches, particularly on the inside of my legs, and no matter how much I scratched I could not get to the itch.

If I gave up my focus of what I wanted my future to be, it would be fatal.

Through it all I knew that I could not give up. If I gave up my focus of what I wanted my future to be, it would be fatal.

Slowly I began to recover some of the feelings in my legs. I have always driven a lot of miles in my work. During this time driving truly became an adventure, especially at night. I learned quickly to pay attention to where my hands were. On one occasion when I was driving home late at night my car started to veer to the right. I knew that I had not moved the steering wheel in that direction and wondered what was wrong with the car. As I looked down on the steering wheel my heart skipped a beat. My hands had fallen from the steering wheel and into my lap without me being aware of it. No more driving tired! I was wide awake for the rest of the trip home.

Over the next few months I regained more coordination and feeling in my body. I noticed that the feeling that was coming back into my hands was different than the feeling had been before I went numb. There was a sense of pressure, but the feeling in my hands was like they were asleep. It was another adjustment.

I laid in bed one evening seeing my beavers working ever-so-diligently working for my benefit. I realized that my outcome might not be completely the same as before the first episode of the MS during the Thanksgiving of 1988. The feeling of loss that I might not ever feel the true touch of my wife's skin again was overwhelming; that holding hands would not be a simple task, because my hand continued to squeeze without me knowing it. At times my wife had to pry our hands apart. Even the basics of holding a glass or cup was changing. If the container was paper, Styrofoam, or aluminum my claw grip would actually crush it. I would not even know that it was happening until the liquid was spilling over my hands.

The losses and adjustments were starting to add up. I had picked up the guitar and drums (they said I was always banging on something) at about age 10 and added the banjo later on. My dad loved playing the guitar, and it was something that we could do together, even though he didn't think Rock & Roll was really music. Every time I placed my fingers on the strings and then looked away the sound was horrible. I looked back at my fingers and saw they had moved without me knowing it. Music has always been very important to me and then, at least for the time being, my ability to produce music was gone. I then remembered that any feeling was better than the prognosis of the neurologist, but experiencing loss is rarely logical.

My boys also didn't like the idea of my not regaining the feeling in my hands. I believed in spanking as a consequence when the boys got in trouble

(OK, I see the e-mails and letters coming now—I've repented). Just before such an event I would tell them, "This is going to hurt you more than it does me," and they knew just what I meant.

As the months passed I continued to see the neurologist. It quickly became very apparent that he was very fond of that round pointy medical instrument that he used on my very first visit. He also added another very technical, highly complex medical device in the array of tests he gave me. It was a pin! He would stick me with the pin and ask if I could feel anything. On my hands, feet, and legs he would stick me. Most of the time I didn't feel anything, but once in a while he did hit a nerve and both of us would jump in surprise. He always said at the end of his exam, "You're doing well," but you still have something (MS).

It occurred to me that I was smart enough to be able to stick myself with a pin, so about six months into the adventure I decided to stop seeing the doctor. Again, this is a decision that I made that I felt was in my best interest. I'm not encouraging anyone that is experiencing any type of illness to stop seeing their doctor or therapist. I was still visualizing my beavers in my brain and since the doctor did not have any specific recommendations to give me, I didn't see any reason to continue.

This is the part of my story that I think is a little mundane and boring. It became such a routine for me to take inventory of my body in the morning. I went through my day at work and participated with my family in the evening and then went to bed at night visualizing the beavers working in my brain.

The progress was slow and there were times I wondered if the benefit was worth the effort. Luckily for me, my wife and I are both very stubborn individuals, and we don't give in very easily. I believe it's important to celebrate the progress of inches as well as miles. The fact that I was still improving was a victory.

Often I'm asked if I ever got discouraged or depressed through this process. "Of course" is always my answer. I'm human just like anyone else.

As a business coach I tell my clients when they get discouraged and want to quit, "Quit, but just don't stop." Keep putting one foot

Quit, but just don't stop.

in front of the other. It doesn't matter how fast we move toward our goals, it matters that we keep moving to our goals. The key is to focus on your desired outcome. The adventure continues.

Action Steps - Chapter 5

Make a list of all the reasons that when you feel discouraged, you're compelled to go on. Dig deep on this one. Look for the emotional ties in relationships, such as doing something for a grandchild.

6

What You Don't Know *Can* Kill You!

I have always enjoyed the movie Fiddler on the Roof. The father's (Tevye) conversations, discussions, and arguments with God are very true to life. In one particular scene he's almost pleading with God that just because he is one of the chosen people, he would like God to bless someone else for a little while, because his blessings are killing him!

That's the way I felt six months after the original diagnosis of MS. Another challenge was just around the corner. For years friends and family had given me grief about my snoring. It had been described many different ways, but it was always non-flattering. A number of years before the diagnosis of MS, a business partner and I had taken a business trip together. He had heard about the stories of my snoring from my wife but dismissed it as a spouse's over exaggeration. Was he in for a big surprise! When we turned off the lights, I went to sleep first. My snoring was so loud that the people in the adjoining room started banging on the wall. Since there was no way for him to get to sleep he decided to get his tape recorder and record me. I had been telling people that it was all in their minds, and that I did not snore any more than anyone else.

The next morning he played the sounds I had made the night before. The best way to describe what I heard is the sounds of a wounded walrus. There were periods of dead silence followed by the gasping and rushing of air as if I had only moments to live if I didn't get more oxygen immediately. The next time

> *The best way to describe what I heard is the sounds of a wounded walrus.*

we traveled together we got separate rooms, located on opposite sides of the hotel.

Sharon had gotten used to finding me sitting straight up in bed fully asleep. She would wake me up enough to have me lay back down, but in a few minutes I would be sitting up again. There would also be long periods of time where I would simply stop breathing, sometimes for up to 40 seconds. The silence would actually wake Sharon, and she would shake me to have me breathe again. She wanted me to go to the doctor and find out what was wrong, but I always brushed off the idea as not being important.

You would think with all these indicators that I would be concerned, but I wasn't. I knew that I woke up tired every morning, but I just thought it was because I was putting in a lot of hours building my business. The kids and I played a game on the way to school every morning. When we stopped at a stoplight I put the car in park and closed my eyes. I immediately fell asleep, and when the light turned green the boys woke me up, and we continued on down the road. You may wonder how many flashing red lights I had to see before I paid attention. That is a good question. Another part of the story, however, was that because of the lack of regenerating sleep I no longer had the ability to make logical and rational decisions. It is very similar to someone that is oxygen deprived. They look fully awake but are unable to connect the dots in any logical way.

> *Part of my thought process was that I had received my quota of bad news for a lifetime. Boy, was I wrong.*

My symptoms from the diagnosis of MS were getting better each week. Part of my thought process was that I had received my quota of bad news for a lifetime. Boy, was I wrong. Finally, my best friend took me aside and asked me why I was playing Russian roulette with my family. He said that I owed it to them to get medically checked out to see what the sleep challenge was.

So I made an appointment with my primary care doctor. When I described the symptoms he made a quick phone call, and I was scheduled for an overnight sleep study the next day. When I asked him what he was looking for, he said I showed all of the signs of having sleep apnea "but not to worry." I'd heard that before!

The next evening I showed up at 10 o'clock to check in to the hospital sleep center. With this being another first, I had no idea what to expect. They took all of the normal vital signs and completed what seemed to be a large amount of paperwork for an overnight test. A nurse then brought me into the room where I would spend the night. It was very bright and full of medical devices and instruments full of red and green flashing lights. I wondered how I would ever get to sleep in such an environment. Over the next half hour or so they attached so many wires to my body that I started to feel like I was part of the machine. I had wires attached to my forehead, chest, arms, and stomach. I also had a strap that went around my chest. At last they said I was ready to go to bed. They reassured me there would be someone all night long monitoring my sleeping. Surprisingly I was able to get to sleep fairly easily and only woke up a few times during the night.

In the morning, a nurse came in to wake me and get me ready to go home. I felt like I finally took a test I could not fail. How could anyone not pass a test when the only requirement was that they fall asleep? I sat in a room and the discharge planning nurse came in. She started by saying that I was not the most severe case of sleep apnea they had ever tested; I was number two. The twist to the story was that number one had died in his sleep, so I was being promoted to number one (I always wanted to be number one in something, but this was getting ridiculous). She said they normally did not send home a continuous positive airway pressure (CPAP) machine with people that had just taken the test at the sleep center, and that they were going to make an exception with me, because they were concerned that I could die before my machine arrived.

> *Who knew that going to sleep could be hazardous to your health?!*

She went on to tell me that the study showed I was expending as much energy every night as a marathon runner did in a race. I was actually waking up more tired in the morning than when I went to bed. Who knew that going to sleep could be hazardous to your health?!

So here I was again with another adjustment. Another loss. Another you've got to be kidding me moment. While I was somewhat relieved to know why I was always so tired, I now had to modify the way I slept. Many people who are prescribed CPAP machines never use them, or use them way too little. They can be uncomfortable and hot. The first night I wore the mask with the CPAP, I knew I had to create another visualization in order to incorporate wearing the mask into my life. This one, though, came to me quicker. If you remember I really love airplanes and the mask resembled a fighter pilot's mask, so you know what I did. I became a fighter pilot every night, flying my jet over my beaver community. Now you *know* I'm weird :-)

This experience, while challenging, was very rewarding. I actually woke up. I had been walking around in a fog without knowing it. I was given another life sentence.

Action Steps - Chapter 6

The question with this chapter can be a little more difficult. My question to you is, "What are you not paying attention to, that you should be?" Many times the things that we do not want to deal with are the very issues that will stop us from receiving our vision.

7

The Machine - Revisited

Over the next five years the symptoms of MS got better and then deteriorated again. About two years after the initial diagnosis I had another major episode, going completely numb from the neck down. I remember the helpless feeling that there was nothing I could do to stop the progressive numbness and thinking, "Oh crap, not again!" There was also something less scary about what was happening to me, because I had gone through it before. Overall, though, anyone that would meet me who did not know my story would not know about the MS diagnosis. At times I was told that I walked deliberately or was a little clumsy when I would walk into a wall or a doorjamb, but they didn't really think anything about it. Part of the reason was that I never took on the identity of having a disability.

An example of that came in 2000 when my youngest son, Chris, and I attended a Tony Robbins nine-day event in Hawaii. I was partnered with a woman from Frankfurt, Germany. Over the nine days we shared a lot of very personal information, and it was a tremendous experience. After arriving home from the event I wrote an article that also included a piece of the MS story.

I received an e-mail from my Robbins partner, and she was very upset. She wanted to know why I had not trusted her enough to share the MS story with her. The truth was that I had not kept the story from her; it just never occurred to me to share it. That week I participated in a number of physical events, including the completion of a 40 foot world-class firewalk and climbing and jumping from a 40 foot telephone pole towards a trapeze bar. I never wanted the diagnosis of the MS to be an excuse that would lead to an "I can't because" response.

The firewalk was a special challenge. I not only had to deal with the fear of getting burned, but also of not falling. There was a part of me that did want to use the "I can't because" card, but I knew that if I used that card it would be very easy to use it again the next time I faced a challenge.

> *I never wanted the diagnosis of the MS to be an excuse that would lead to an "I can't because" response.*

It takes a few hours to prepare to do the firewalk. We actually went out to "meet the fire" and it was so hot that you could only stand next to it for a few seconds. When I got in line to take my turn, I remember finding a point of light beyond the fire. I focused intently on the light, and when I was tapped on the shoulder signaling that it was my time to go, I was ready. It was only one step into the unknown! You have a deep sense of needing to run before you get burned, but I had great instructors and knew that it was only by taking deliberate steps, one at a time, that I would be able to make it the entire 40 feet. The entire experience lasts less than a minute, but there are times when it seems like everything stands still, and then you have a sensation that time accelerated. I made it to the end without even a singed hair on my legs. What a rush!

The firewalk reinforced my belief that even though an obstacle was before me I could adjust my circumstances and create an outcome that I desired. It would not be my last opportunity to test that belief, but I'm getting ahead of myself.

There is an old saying that when you come to an obstacle that blocks your path you have many options. You can go over it, under it, around it, or through it. Even with all of those options you still have one more. You may decide that the foot of the mountain was your destination all along. I look at the obstacles that the symptoms of the MS have given me as opportunities. Yes, there are many times when I really wish that I had a few less of those opportunities to deal with. It can become very tiresome, but again it's a small price to pay for a life sentence.

A friend of mine in Texas, who was a life insurance underwriter, called me one day. He said, "Gary, you don't act normal." Well he wasn't the first person who ever told me that. He went on to say that I didn't act normal for someone who was diagnosed with Multiple Sclerosis, and that he wanted me to go and have another MRI. Oh goody! Just what I wanted to hear. I get to go revisit that machine again. He thought maybe in the original diagnosis someone had made a mistake.

This time I went to the MS center in Denver with a new neurologist. The doctor agreed with my friend, and we scheduled my new test. I was pleased that in the last five years they had moved the MRI from a tractor-trailer to a hospital facility. As far as I could tell that was the only difference in the experience. I remember the first neurologist telling me not to get my hopes up, that, in his opinion, my future had a 10 year expiration date on it. Yet here I was taking another MRI with a different doctor, saying the first test could be wrong. Could it really be true that I was dealing with something completely different for the last five years and, if so, what was it?

The day of the test came and, having been through the exam before, I knew the routine. During the four segments of the MRI, I again visualized and took a trip to Hawaii. The test itself somehow didn't seem quite as intimidating as it had been in my first experience. One of my Gary-isms is "the first time always is." You may be saying duh, that was really profound. It really is, because what I mean is that your first time in anything, you don't know what that experience will bring. The fear that can be felt in a first-time event is, then, normal.

I was really looking forward to getting the test results later in the week with my new neurologist. I knew that he would have good news for me. The time finally came for me to get the results of my new MRI.

When the doctor came into the room he had a very puzzled look on his face. He held in his hand the film from the first MRI from five years before and the film of the recent MRI. He looked at me and said, "I really don't understand what I'm looking at from these two tests." The first test clearly showed the white specks on the brain, indicating the lesions. The second test showed that 95% of those lesions, which are scar tissue, were gone. He looked at me and said that this simply could not have happened. He had seen MS patients go into remission and have the deterioration in the patient's brain slow or stop altogether, but never had he seen a case where the scar tissue simply seemed to disappear.

I asked him what this really all meant for me. He looked at me like I had asked a very silly question and said, "Oh, you still have MS, and I want to see you every six months to track your progression." I know the disappointment showed on my face.

The doctor then wanted to know what kind of treatment I had been receiving over the last five years. I told him that I had decided not to go the steroid route and shared with him that I had created a visualization using beavers in my brain to patch up the myelin sheath. Now he gave me that you've got to be kidding look and said that I had to be doing something medically to get these types of results. He couldn't come to grips with the idea that my visualization of beavers in my brain might actually have worked. I left his office that day and haven't been back since.

Could it really be true that 95% of the lesions on my brain were gone? If they were gone why was I still experiencing the symptoms that, by now, I had grown somewhat accustomed to? I then remembered something else that I tell many of my business coaching clients: "We don't always have to understand it, we just have to embrace it." I still had my life sentence, and my beavers were still working three shifts around the clock. I had my focus on the future with my oldest son going into high school, and I was getting closer to that 100th birthday party.

So why was I bummed? I think the answer to that question came down to this. I wanted to be normal, just like everyone else. So here was another life lesson I got to explore. The next logical question to me was, what is normal? The answer surprised me. It was to blend in. If you told anyone around me my objective was to blend into my surroundings, they would not have believed you. I had played sports in high school and was a drummer. I ran singing groups and a little theater in college. I had even driven a destruction derby car when I was 17 years old. I had very definite opinions about most things and was normally not bashful in sharing them.

> *I wanted to be normal, just like everyone else.*

But this was different. This was tied to my male ego. Today Multiple Sclerosis is considered an invisible disability, but it becomes visible at the most inopportune times. I didn't want to seem clumsy or awkward and despised the feelings of dependence in the simple things such as buttoning a shirt. I was grateful to have been given a life sentence twice, and I knew my next big milestone would be the 10 year anniversary of the first diagnosis.

Action Steps - Chapter 7

The last time that you received news that was opposite than that which you wanted, how did you handle the news? This is an important question because there are times when we receive disappointing news, and we might interpret that news with a story that may not have any basis in fact.

8

The Anniversary

Thanksgiving 1998 was the 10 year anniversary. Surprisingly, it came and went without much notice. In the last 10 years there had been two major episodes. I had lost and regained the ability to walk (almost) in a straight line. My ability to write slowly came back. As I relearned to write there were many humorous moments, particularly when I would go to sign my name at a checkout counter. Because I had lost the dexterity in my fingers I would grab the pen and put it in the middle of my fist. My best attempts at writing my name at times were no more than scribbles. I sometimes got the look from the checkout person of what was that I had just written? So I would look them straight in the eye and say, "It sucks to be famous," and then they would wonder who I really was.

> *I would look them straight in the eye and say, "It sucks to be famous," and then they would wonder who I really was.*

I was determined not to allow the inconvenience of the symptoms that persisted to deter me from living life to the fullest. In August of 1993 I climbed my first two 14,000 foot mountains here in Colorado. By no means was I the fastest person on the mountain that day, but I may have been the most focused. And I'll tell you, the view from the top is awesome. When you're on top of a 14,000 foot peak, and you see airplanes flying lower than where you're standing, it's an experience you will not soon forget. Another one of the life lessons I have learned through this experience is to compete only with myself. When I compete with myself I will always win, but when I compete with someone else one of us has to lose. The victory is in completing the race, not always coming in first.

My sons, Matt and Chris, also gave me opportunities to show that I could take on virtually any challenge. For Father's Day my son, Chris, decided to give me a present. He told me that he wanted to be there when I opened it up, and as that was a little unusual I started to wonder what he had in mind.

If any of you Dads out there have teenage sons, you know that there would be three things to be concerned about here. First, that he knew it was Father's Day. Second, then he had a present for me. Third, that he wanted to be there when I opened the present. Father's Day finally came and Chris handed me a shoebox. I opened it ever so carefully and when I peeked inside I saw one of those bungee tiedown cords. Chris had been asking to go camping with me (my idea of camping is staying at the Holiday Inn), and I knew that I wanted to build some neat memories with him before he went to college.

I took a deep breath and was about to say where would you like to go camping when I caught a twinkle in Chris's eyes. At that moment I knew I wasn't going camping—I was going bungee jumping!

About a year later, Matt, Chris's older brother, was moving with his wife, Kelly, to Davenport, Iowa. A couple of weeks before they were to leave he gave me a call. He told me that before they left he wanted to share another experience with me—to Fly On A Trapeze! Again I had an opportunity to meet a challenge. My concern on the trapeze was not the height (although it was a little intimidating), it was not knowing if, when I left the platform, I would be able to hold on to the bar because I had very little feeling or sensation in my hands.

I again wanted to build special memories with Matt and Kelly before they left, but also my male ego didn't want to look foolish. (Both Matt and Kelly taught circus dance at a camp in Pennsylvania and were very accomplished on the trapeze.) I remember thinking, as I was on the platform about ready to take that step into thin air, that this was no different than facing the other challengers in my life. It was about being extremely focused on the task at hand.

Both the experience of the bungee jump and trapeze were exhilarating and extremely freeing. To engage in both events all it came down to was taking one step into the unknown. Wow, what a life lesson. I am always grateful for the opportunities to test my ability to face a challenge. Thanks, Kids!

In 2000 I had the opportunity to meet and work with John Gray, author of *Men are from Mars, Women are from Venus.* In a speech, I had heard John talk about working with individuals that had been given the diagnosis of Multiple Sclerosis and wanted to get his take on the dynamics of the illness.

John explained to me that he had never worked with a MS patient that was not what he called "a receptor," a person who receives energy from other people. The beliefs of these people were that they needed to take in the negative energy around them, so it would not hurt anyone else.

The problem with that, John explained, was that as you take in that negative energy and you don't release it, you start to go numb to your surroundings. This would not only affect your physical health but also your relationships and your ability in business. The ultimate numbness would be death. He suggested that I create a visualization that allowed me to still deal with people and their problems but to create a process that also allowed me to let it go.

Living in Colorado we experience a lot of lightning. For some reason as John was speaking to me I saw a picture of a lightning rod. Lightning rods draw in energy and then disperse it into the ground where it cannot hurt anyone. I loved that idea. I didn't have to change who I was in dealing with people from all over the world with many challenges. As a business coach "that includes life" (I don't believe that we can separate our personal lives from our business life), I was still able to be intensely involved in the process of my clients but by redirecting and dispersing the energy I could now facilitate a positive conclusion for myself, as well as my clients.

As time went on, I started to tell my story more publicly. When I was originally diagnosed I owned a financial planning firm. Because of the sensitivity of the nature of the industry I didn't want to alarm my clients that a doctor had given me a relatively short time to live. I didn't think this would be beneficial to my practice. By not openly sharing my story I was also able to more effectively focus on what I believed was my future. As time went on, however, and more people knew some of what my story was, I felt more compelled to share bits and pieces that would help others dealing with adversity to have hope.

My first opportunity to share my complete story came in 2003. Joe Vitale, the author of *Attractor Factor*, sent me an e-mail requesting anyone who had dealt and overcome an adversity to submit the story to him to possibly be included in his upcoming book. At first I was really reluctant to put my story down on paper but decided that if I could benefit just one person it would be worth the exposure.

I wrote up the "Reader's Digest condensed" version of my experience and sent it off to Joe, and heard absolutely nothing back. I figured that my story had not been accepted and thought nothing more about it, until I received an e-mail 10 months later that was very strange.

In the subject line of the e-mail there were symbols that look like hieroglyphics (the kind you see when it's a Viagra e-mail—you guys know what I mean!) So I opened it. ☺! In the text of the e-mail the writer was telling me part of my story. This was really weird because, to my knowledge, I had not published anything about my experience. Because what he was telling me was accurate, I responded back to him, even though his English grammar was very poor. I asked him where he had read about me. He responded back that he had read my story in one of Joe Vitale's new books. Now he had my attention. I was so excited about the prospect of being in one of Joe's books that I jumped into my car and went immediately down to look at the local bookstore. I knew *Attractor Factor Two* had just been released. I thought it would be really cool if I had been included in the book. I didn't want to get too excited, but when I finally found a copy, it only took a few minutes to search all of the pages for my story. I wasn't there. I was disappointed to say the least. But where could my new e-mail contact have read about my story? I sent another e-mail telling him that I could not find my story in *Attractor Factor Two*. He responded, "Of course not, it's in a second book that Joe Vitale just released called *Expect Miracles*." When I found a copy of *Expect Miracles* my story **was** in it. Two pages' worth, with my name and website address listed at the end of my story. Wow, that's how my new e-mail friend had been able to find me.

I was also curious to know where he lived and, as it turned out, it was in the Ukraine. That also explained his poor English grammar. Since that time I've had many e-mail contacts from people all over the world, many of whom know someone or are dealing with Multiple Sclerosis or some other debilitating disease. I feel very blessed to be able to reach back out to them, and to share my experience with them. I started to feel guilty that I had not shared my story sooner. Why had I waited so long? A partial answer is that I didn't think I had done anything special. I'm just an ordinary guy who made a decision to live.

I have found that as I tell my story, others I come in contact with seem to have permission to share their personal stories as well. We all have a story that is valuable. What is yours?

> *I'm just an ordinary guy who made a decision to live.*

I believe that we are all on the same path, just at different mile markers. In a sense we can all become guides to those that come behind us. As we travel the path, at times the trail seems to disappear. This can give us a feeling like we're lost, even though we are still on the right path. On mountain trails when the path seems to disappear, stacks of rocks are used, called cairns. These rock piles are spaced apart just far enough that the hiker doesn't lose the trail and get lost. There have been many times during my adventure with the diagnosis of Multiple Sclerosis that I felt like I was on the wrong trail. For whatever reason, my ultimate vision that I saw for myself became obscured. These were the times I felt most afraid, because I didn't want to make a wrong step. The question that allowed me to continue many times was simply "What is my next step?" This question allowed me to refocus on what was right before me, which allowed me to get beyond my fear and keep my momentum. Sometimes it's the simple questions that give us the greatest answers.

I found that one of the hardest situations to deal with were the ones that dealt with loss. I had started to play the drums in my early teens but had drifted away from playing after getting married. About 10 years ago I was asked to play for a praise band at the church I was attending. I knew I wanted to, but I also knew that with the limited feelings in my hands it could be challenging to know when I had control of the drumsticks and when I didn't.

All of the macho feelings came rushing back in, even though I really love music. I didn't want to embarrass myself by throwing my drumstick and hitting someone (which was a very real possibility). I argued with myself for the next couple of months but finally said yes. It was one of the best decisions I ever made. Yes, I have had challenges playing the drums, but it has given me the stimulus to be creative. Because drumsticks are smooth they were constantly flying out of my hands (after a performance people would come up, and congratulate me on my fancy stick work.

What they didn't know was I had not intended for the stick to fly out of my hand, and that I was just reaching out to catch it to be able to continue to play!). I rubbed the sticks with sandpaper, wore gloves, but nothing seemed to help. Then it came to me that I could use double-sided sticky tape to wrap around the drumsticks. It worked! I now get offers to play almost every week.

So was my original sense of loss, my belief that I could no longer play the drums, a positive or negative event? Over the past 22 years I have found it helpful not to judge events as good or bad. The event just "is." I look at them as being different, even when I'm experiencing a physical challenge. This is more than just saying words to fool myself into accepting a particular situation. It's embracing the belief that I cannot control what happens to me but, rather, I can only control my reaction to what happens to me. This belief has served me very well and, if you embrace this belief, it will work for you, too.

Remember life is an adventure. I would like to encourage you to come along with me and "enjoy the ride."

Action Steps Chapter 8

Are you ready to share your story with other people? If you are, this would be a great time to write an article showcasing your story. What are the major points of your story that would be of the biggest help to someone reading the article? Don't worry about being perfect, just share.

9

The Final Chapter

The final chapter is not an accurate title. Obviously I'm still here and still getting into trouble, much to my delight. I have started telling people at my speeches that "I am the best looking dead man walking they have ever seen." That may sound a little morbid to you, but through this experience I have come to embrace both life and death. Because of not hiding from the reality that we will all die at some point, I have been able to understand time in a different way. Time is an asset, just like money. The only difference is that when you spend time there is no way to get it back. Once it's gone it's gone. I remember when I was in my 20s, like many people, thinking that the time I had on this Earth was unlimited.

So every day I have the opportunity to decide how I will invest the 24 hours that have been deposited into my life account. Again, instead of looking at activities as not being good or bad or right or wrong, I ask

Is this activity leading me towards my vision or away from my vision?

myself the question "is this activity leading me towards my vision or away from my vision?" This leaves me free to be very creative and deliberate in the way I spend my time. I haven't always had this perspective, though, in regards to time.

An example of one of my challenges with time revolves around TV. As a baby boomer growing up in the 50s and 60s television was not only new, it was a status symbol. In the home that I grew up in the TV was literally on 24 hours a day, seven days a week, 365 days a year. I even remember as a kid, coming into the living room and seeing the TV on with the test pattern glowing in the dark. Now, I'm not suggesting that everyone get rid of their television sets, but what I came to realize is that I was using TV as a way of escaping my reality. I'm using my experience with TV only to illustrate one of my roadblocks I found that prevented me from receiving my desired outcomes. Don't get me wrong, I still watch TV, but I watch it now consciously by making a deliberate decision to do so.

On one particular trip, I was sitting in an airport and thinking how I always felt there was just not enough time. I decided to list all of my activities in any given week, with an estimated amount of time given to each activity. The results took me by surprise. It showed that I was literally spending 15 to 20 hours per week more than I had to spend. One of the stories I had been telling myself was that I did not have time to go to the gym and work out, even though I knew that going to the gym would help my body repair itself. Because of that belief my weight had increased to 249 pounds, and since I am not six foot three, I was not in shape (as of this writing, I'm happy to share that my current weight is 214 pounds). So, why am I sharing these details with you? Because, I want you to know that it's the little details that provide you with the big results.

From the very beginning of the adventure with Multiple Sclerosis and sleep apnea, I knew I wanted to have a balanced life. What that means to me is that I have a great family life, a spiritual connection with God, a body full of energy and vitality, and a creative and vibrant business outlet that provides the resources for my family and me. Have I always been able to achieve the desired results? No, but I have never totally lost my momentum on my road to triumph.

About 10 years ago I had a very impactful dream. I played football in high school and have always loved the sport. In my dream I saw myself in the backfield, which was a strange place for me to be, since I was a defensive end, but as I looked ahead at the line I also saw myself in my normal position. Even though in the dream I knew this wasn't quite right I assumed that somehow it was normal. Just before the ball was snapped, for some reason, I took a quick look into the grandstands. What I saw was me looking back at me. Weird! As I looked back to the line to engage in the next play a James Earl Jones voice came from above (James Earl Jones sure gets around a lot). The deep, resonant, calming voice asked, "Are you a participant or are you a spectator?" This confused me because obviously I was on the field engaged in a sport I loved, so I dismissed the voice.

Again, I turned back to the play and again that James Earl voice asked more deliberately, "Are you a participant or are you a spectator, it's your choice!" My choice, what was he talking about? Then my dream came into clear focus. I had just seen myself playing on both sides of the ball as well as in the stands. In my dream, and later I realized in my life, I had not made a clear choice of where my life was going to take me.

> *Are you a participant or are you a spectator, it's your choice!*

What was comforting and a little disturbing at the same time was that I did have a choice—to either be a participant or a spectator, and it was truly all right either way. The bottom line, though, was that I did have to make a choice. If I chose to make no choice, it was actually a choice of being a spectator. Then I woke up in a cold sweat. It was about two in the morning, and I wasn't able to go back to sleep. I realized that, for the last 12 years, while I was progressing with my life, I was not fully living life. I had toyed around with the idea of sharing my story and insights with audiences around the world but had done nothing to put that idea into action. Another one of my Gary-isms is that "Our worst day is the day that we meet the man or woman we could have been."

So I decided to truly be a participant. Within three weeks I held my first public seminar around the psychology and emotions we have with money. I completed and released my first e-book *Financial Magic* with the patience and help from my family. I reengaged in playing the drums that energized and revitalized my soul. This book and my book *On Purpose Results* are other results of that decision.

I have had the opportunity to speak nationally and internationally to thousands of people. If I had not made the definite decision to take action I would never have had this opportunity. I always receive so much more from hearing the stories of those individuals that have come to hear me. It constantly reminds me that we all have a story to share (if you or anyone you know would like me to come and speak, my contact information is at the back of this book).

As I wrote at the beginning of this chapter, this is not the final chapter. It is only the next chapter in the rest of my life. The road from adversity to triumph is a road that we are all on, just at different mile markers. My hope and prayer is that no matter where you are on that road, you will not allow anything to get in the way of your destiny. At birth you have been given everything you need to finish your trip. Sometimes we don't know where all of those resources are, but all you have to do is "ask" and the answer to *your next step* will appear.

Thank you for taking and sharing this part of my journey with me.

Action Steps - Chapter 9

What is your vision for your future? Go 3, 5, and 10 years or longer into your future and envision exactly what it will be like. Don't become discouraged if this question takes a little longer, because I find most people are out of practice in this exercise. Remember to make it as real as possible.

10

Epilogue

As I have captured in this book the events of the last 22 years of my life, it was more difficult than I thought it would be. There were parts of my story that even I had forgotten. The telling of my losses would actually take me back to some of the raw emotions I felt during the original experience. It was as if somehow I had found a time machine, and I found myself back in 1988 at Thanksgiving. I have been asked if writing this book was worth it, and I have to say a heartfelt, Yes it was! It has given me the opportunity to re-experience the events and decisions of my past that have made me the person I am today.

As I came to the closing chapter I also found it difficult to stop writing (which is unique for me, because I am a speaker that had to become a writer). I wanted the last words in this book to leave you with a sense of hope, inspiration, and direction. Therefore, I decided to boil down the book to three suggestions.

First, create and hold fast to your clear **Vision**. Having a clear vision is much more than just setting goals for yourself. It's going into your future and making that future so real that you can see it, taste it, and feel it. Once you have developed that picture, you

Create and hold fast to your clear Vision.

can tie yourself to it with elastic rope. Your vision will serve as your anchor that you can trust. It has to be crystal clear, and it has to be personally yours. By stretching that vision and bringing that picture of your experience back to your present situation you will create what I call "your personal déjà vu." If you do this, you will be pulled to your vision. I have heard it described in the past as "telling the truth in advance." What you are waiting for is time to pass for your future vision to become your reality. This picture of your vision is what I suggest you focus on.

Second, uncover what your **Beliefs** are. Our beliefs are what run our subconscious. In my book *On Purpose Results* I make the bold statement that 99% of the results we have now in our lives are from decisions that are on purpose. They are either consciously on purpose or subconsciously on purpose. The problem is that most of those decisions are made in our subconscious. That's why it's critical to know what your personal beliefs are.

One very important belief to look at is "do you deserve?" The belief that a person does not deserve is the most common and devastating belief that I have found that my business coaching clients have. That one belief of not deserving is poison to relationships, building businesses and careers, and any meaningful relationship to a higher power. Ask yourself what you believe about money, love, acceptance, deserving, God, or any other topic you feel connected to. As you ask these questions, it is very likely that you will be very uncomfortable in the process, but you will enjoy the end result.

Third, **have courage, develop a plan, and launch**. One of my childhood heroes was John Wayne. I have watched most of his movies and it didn't matter if he was in an Indian war, a World War II battle of Iwo Jima, or was engaged in an aerial dogfight with the Flying Tigers, he showed no fear. I embraced what I thought was the underlying message of his movies, to be courageous was to have no fear.

Through my experience with the diagnosis of Multiple Sclerosis I have changed my definition of courage. I have learned that fear is normal, natural, and needed. My new definition of courage is "Action in the presence of fear."

> *My new definition of courage is "Action in the presence of fear."*

After one of my speeches, one of the individuals in the audience came up to me saying my definition of fear really connected for him. Part of his story was that he was part of the invasion on Omaha Beach during D-Day. He told me there was not a single person in his landing craft in the invasion that day that was not afraid. The difference of living or dying that day many times was determined by what action each man took in the presence of fear. He saw and knew that if he froze and did nothing he would surely be killed. He also knew that if he moved forward and took action to get out of the landing craft and on to the beach he might also be killed, but that was the only way he also had a chance to live. Wow, what a story!

Launching by taking action is always fear producing, because no one has a crystal ball of what the actual outcome will be. That is why developing and taking action on a plan is so important. Your plan is your roadmap that allows you to know if you're on course or not. This can be the formula for addressing any situation in your life.

When the first neurologist told me his belief was that I would be dead or in a wheelchair within 10 years, that was fear producing. I could have chosen not to move and to accept his prognosis. I knew I had to take on a different belief and create a vivid vision for my future. Without this third step of having courage, developing a plan, and launching, I know that I would not be here today.

I know that anyone reading this book can have the life of their dreams. The prize at the end of the day often doesn't come to the strongest or the swiftest but, instead, comes to that person that chooses never to give up.

So I have come to the conclusion of *Into the Night*, but I will not say goodbye, only so long. I hope that we have an opportunity at some point to have a formal introduction where I can learn what your personal "Road from Adversity to Triumph" story is.

To your success,

Gary

A Note from Gary

I hope this book has helped you in your own personal journey. If you would like to share how this book as made a difference in your life, please write to me. I am always excited to read your personal stories. Send your letters or e-mails to:

Gary Barnes International
3500 S. Wadsworth Blvd.
Suite 203
Denver, CO 80235
e-mail: Gary@GaryBarnesInternational.com
website: www.GaryBarnesInternational.com

A possible next step with Gary

Gary has created a remarkable program called On a Purpose Results. The On Purpose Results E-Course is a 13-week course designed to give you the mindset tools and techniques to make you more flexible, more agile, more confident, and more successful. It lets you "be your own coach." To have more fun with your business. To expand your mindset. And to make the world better while improving yourself. Go to www.onpurposeresults.com to learn more.

To your success!

If you enjoyed
Into the Night
Gary Barnes is The Ideal Professional Speaker for Your Next Event!

"The Traction Coach"

Gary Barnes is an International Speaker as seen on ABC, CBS, NBC & FOX , will leave your audience laughing and learning. An author, business coach, and professional speaker for over 25 years, Gary's high energy and humor will entertain, inspire AND deliver a message that is dynamic, impactful and FUN! Gary uses the power of story to help his audiences take charge of their lives—to ignite their dreams and release their blocks so they can reach their own personal summits.

Gary believes anyone can lead an empowered life, no matter what their circumstances are. He has built three successful businesses from the ground up. He also understands dealing with adversity-he has fought life-threatening illness and won. He believes that your worst day is the day you meet the man or woman you could have been. It's a choice.

Gary's Most Requested Programs
(Engaging, Deeply Touching, Hilarious)

- **Into the Night** – The Road from Adversity to Triumph
- **Take a Flying Leap** - How to Prosper in a Difficult Economy
- **Maximize Your Business Now** – with On Purpose Results!

If you would like to know more about booking Gary for a keynote, breakout or workshop, please contact our office by calling 303-989-0066 or toll-free 1-877-276-7102.

You may also e-mail your questions to:
Info@GaryBarnesInternational.com.

Share This Book!

Quantity discounts of this book are available.
Call us for more information and a quotation.
Personalized autographed copies are also available.

Get Rid y old
Thads old - In new -Good Bye!

Take away Room4 Conscience
#1 impossibility - no real bt
2 possibty - reduced
3. probability - learny frund
4. Inevitabilty →

CPSIA information can be obtained at www.ICGtesting.com
Printed in the USA
266757BV00001B/1/P

9 780983 763000